SWEET TREATS FOR KIDS

Suzanna Malinosky

Contents

Chapter One

INTRODUCTION

Anxiousness is a part of my nature, and I can't help it. The more often I can lose myself in the joys of kitchen work, the more likely I am to keep myself busy, tinker with new ideas, and keep myself busy. However, I must say that after the publication of my first book, BabyCakes, I was almost entirely exhausted. After a long day at work, I'd be too fatigued to finish pulling off my shoes and socks before collapsing on the couch. My proudest moment left me immobilised, despite the fact that I am a lifelong runner. Nothing felt right.

However, after a short time, a familiar sensation took over. I began to imagine novel textures and flavour combinations while snoozing in bed each morning. It didn't take me long to start perusing my local grocery and specialty store aisles for new foodstuffs, scrutinising the labels for ingredients and making quick purchases. My brain was racing to the point of a nightmare while I slept. Billboard, rack, and sky colour combinations inspired me to create new colour schemes and textures. When I went shopping, I bought products that I couldn't eat because of my gluten allergy so that I could crack them open, study the insides, and generally make a mess wherever I went.

A few weeks later, I was entirely engulfed in a state of agitation. When I figured out how to make the BabyCakes NYC chocolate-chip cookie work in 2005, I had a similar reaction. I found the inner workings of my cornbread recipe in 2006 when I finally found it. It became crystal evident at that moment: the arrival of a whole new formula was imminent.

Something bold but simple, noble but unapologetically normal: a plain donut covered in chocolate.

My doughnut was vegan and gluten-free so I melted chocolate on top before baking. This one is a lot better than the prior one. The second one was a little less awful, but still awful. It everything came together on the third try. Now, it's no exaggeration to say that BabyCakes NYC was forever altered on that day. Despite the fact that the cupcake, my firstborn's favourite, was tossed, I won't go into detail about it here. You won't find a single cupcake recipe or cupcake reference in these pages after this point in the story of the book you're currently holding. It's as simple as the creation of the first donut. That's up to you, my friends.

After the donut was invented, a slew of other classic products began to emerge. Suddenly, I had a recipe for the pancake, the undisputed hero of my youth. Then came the waffles. Re-creating these timeless recipes in a vegan, gluten-free, health-minded manner steamrolled into six months' worth of absolute chaos inside the BabyCakes NYC test kitchen. My baking team were concerned and perhaps annoyed, but I don't think they were willing to admit it since they were too weirded out by my obsessional attention.

I carried on as if nothing had happened. However, as you'll see, this collection of recipes was more about expanding on what I already understood about my key ingredients than it was about figuring out how to get them to work together. What I hope you learned from the first book or will learn from this one is that once you've mastered your vegan and gluten-free pantry, the sky is the limit when it comes to what you can bake with them.

The recipes in this book draw heavily on the knowledge gained from the prior book. Repetitive material will not be included in this guidebook. You should not be concerned if you lack the requisite level of inventiveness and affection; I will do my best to simplify and get right to the point in the event that you lack these qualities. As a last resort, don't forget that most of what I covered in my first book can be obtained online at a variety of locations. We will all come out of this relatively undamaged if we work together.

For those who have yet to meet my magical assistants, I hope you've seen them in action while making BabyCakes at either my New York or Los Angeles bakeries. While I might be categorised as a meticulous, recipe-oriented baker, no one could ever accuse me of being overly flamboyant in the kitchen. I'm not a fan of overly-detailed decorations or elaborate sugar sculptures. In terms of design, I strive for simplicity—plainness, if you will. Complications are better left in the batter, in my opinion.

Snacks and treats that are generally out of reach for people with vegan, celiac, or other dietary restrictions have been celebrated in this book. Those emotional classics, which we typically admire in the bakery window but never purchase, are about to enter our lives for the first time this year. Things like Wonder Buns, Thin Mints, and S'Mores are all here, as are Hamentaschen and five different kinds of doughnut. As a last resort, I whipped up some of my favourite savoury recipes, including an onion-cheddar crepe, a vegetable tart, and an amazingly convenient granola. Even if there is always space for improvement, I am constantly hungry.

While the first book provided an introduction to vegan, gluten-free, and agave-based diets, the second is a comprehensive guide.

It is a compilation of humorous treats to help you explore your culinary horizons. It is refreshing to see so many of them being so straightforward. It's a good thing that the complexity of flavour and texture aren't overlooked. You'll have to put in some effort, but I'll be there to support you the whole way.

That's right, there's the work to do. The elements that make baking almost inhumanly frustrating also make it unbelievably satisfying, as you know all too well. To get the sweet pieces beneath your nails and burn batches and listen to your favourite music far too loud is what it's all about here. When it comes to food, it's all about nibbling as you go and testing out new recipes and aprons. A sense of calm and serenity is at the heart of this project. When you have the best time of your life, you collapse to the ground in a fit of hysterics because you can't stop crying. When the timer shakes off the table and lands on the floor, you know it's time. That moment when you realise just how much effort you've put into something, or how perfectly you've done it. The goal is to make everyone around you, even those you don't know well, feel joyous and enthused about something you've never done before.

Additionally, I work as a baker. Every day, I remind myself that I'm one of the luckiest girls in the planet. My greatest want is to be able to share with you some of the incredible riches I've been blessed with as a result of writing this book.

TOOLS, GUIDELINES, AND INGREDIENTS: A REVIEW

Prior to getting started, let's go through the Three Commandments of Cooking, which can be found in any cookbook. If you have the original BabyCakes book, you may be keeping your loved ones awake at night with the following refrain:

Before you begin, take sure to thoroughly read the recipe.

Find and prepare the ingredients you'll need.

Get it right the first time! Make sure you follow the directions to the letter.

Here at BabyCakes NYC, we utilise only the best ingredients to make our cakes, just as you would get in any of your favourite restaurants. At a tremendous cost, everything we use in the bakery now was procured through imbalanced chequebooks, misplaced online orders, and endless scouting of exquisite food markets. Yes, you'll have to deal with some costliness in some of the dishes, and I'm sure I could make some adjustments that would be less expensive. But I will not. In the end, you'd be furious with me.

Due to the variances in water supplies and oven temperatures, as well as variations in the ingredients our suppliers were delivering, we had to make some adjustments to several of our recipes when we established our Los Angeles BabyCakes NYC location. Despite the fact that these in-

If you're cooking in Denver, Colorado, for example, even recipes that have been rigorously tested may require minor adjustments. (I've also been advised that altitude is a factor.) Then again, who knows? Let's all agree to follow the rules while yet being flexible in the kitchen.

One thing to keep in mind: All of the recipes below require dry measuring cups. For maximum scooping, they're usually made of stainless steel and feature long, flat handles that fit snugly together. When it comes to liquid measurements, how about that Pyrex measuring cup you've been using so much lately? If you can, keep it as far away from children and pets as possible.

You'll need to read these additional important tips and tidbits before continuing:

This recipe calls for refined coconut oil in many instances. In order to get accurate measurements, you must first melt your coconut oil.

2. Ensure that your measurements are accurate. Use a dry cup measure to scoop and level the flour. It's important that you get every last drop of liquid out of the cup when you're

measuring oils, milks, or agave nectar. Fruit purees and other liquids that can be poured are the same.

Unless you're following these instructions, don't mess around with substitutes or off-brand ingredients. You're just asking for trouble if you do that. See if you can find and utilise any of the brands I've listed here and elsewhere, like as on the bakery's website and in a broader list from the last book.

Because every oven cooks at a different rate, I've learned this the hard way. Before removing anything from the oven, stick a toothpick into the centre and make sure it comes out clean. For the best baking results, use an oven thermometer.

To prevent them from falling, DO NOT TOUCH YOUR CAKES BEFORE THEY ARE HALF DONE.

In order to accurately measure your food, you need to use special measuring spoons, not the ones you use to mix coffee or consume ice cream.

Call a few close pals for moral support if you start to lose hope.

Ingredients

You already know this from the previous page, but just to be sure, I'll go over it again: the key to any successful meal preparation is using high-quality ingredients. The following are my personal picks for the greatest vegan and gluten-free products on the market today—the absolute must-haves for most of the recipes on this site. The Glossary at the conclusion of this book contains a list of other items that you'll need, but for which the label on the bottle or bag is less significant. These are the brands we use at BabyCakes NYC and the ones that were used to test the recipes in this book, but you are free to use other brands.

Flours made by Bob's Red Mill are gluten-free.

Even though I've said it a gazillion times before, I think it's worth saying again: Everything from their All Purpose Gluten-Free Baking Flour to their Garbanzo and Fava Flour to their baking soda is my favourite. If you've ever baked with substitute ingredients, you'll know how important uniformity is. Note to those with nut allergies: This gluten-free flour is manufactured on the same machinery as almonds and hazelnuts. ′ However, Bob's does all it can to prevent cross-contamination. Each batch of flour is put through a thirty-pound test bag to ensure that all of the nut remnants have been removed from the machinery. Instead of throwing away this perfectly edible flour, Bob's provides it to charitable organisations like animal shelters for free! The milling of gluten-free flour begins when the philanthropic work has been completed. Whether or whether you are comfortable with this is entirely up to you.

Daiya's Dairy-Free Vegan Cheese

This is a vegan, gluten-free cheese that melts like butter and tastes fantastic without the use of preservatives or artificial chemicals. This cake has a base made of tapioca and arrowroot, which are both authorised by BabyCakes NYC.

Enjoy Life's chocolate chip cookies

Finally, I've found a vegan, gluten-free, and dairy-free chocolate that I love! It has a strong, but not overpowering, flavour that may be used in any recipe. It is also free of any trace of soy or nuts.

Unscented Coconut Oil by Omega Nutrition, a 100 percent organic product

Coconut oil is rich in omega-3 fatty acids, has a high concentration of lauric acid, and stores as energy rather than fat. Despite its high price, it's a necessary evil.

Our baking is enhanced by the buttery taste of this brand of odourless coconut oil, but it doesn't overwhelm the flavour of the other ingredients. You can even get scented coconut oil if you're a fanatic about the flavour; however, only use refined oil and heat it up first before using it in a dish.

Light Agave Nectar Organic Nectars

Many agave nectar suppliers have recently been found to be cutting their agave nectars with corn syrup! The answer is emphatically no: Agaves are not to be trifled with. Agave salmiana, a native of Mexico, is used to make the low-glycemic nectar sold by Organic Nectars. Using it in place of honey, corn syrup, and vegan sugar will make your baked goods taste better than the originals. This is the greatest agave nectar I've tried, and I've tried a lot.

Vanilla Singing Dog by Singing Dog

As a result of the purity and flavour of this fair trade vanilla, I've decided to utilise it in all of my BabyCakes locations. Every recipe in these pages can be completed with a single bottle of wine.

Crème Ricemellow is the specialty of Suzanne's Specialties.

A marshmallow substitute is something completely new to me, so finding Suzanne's Specialties' Ricemellow Crème so early on in my search was a huge relief. Please be aware, however, that because this product contains soy protein, it will only be available at my dinner parties and not in my bakeries.

Tools

Last time around, I urged you to get your hands on a wide variety of culinary implements and gadgets. I'm going to presume that many of these are already in your possession, so I won't burden you with a list of them. When it comes to mixing up huge amounts, you've probably got a good supply of glass bowls of all sizes. You already have a whisk, a food processor, a rubber spatula, and toothpicks. Many of the recipes in this book require a few more ingredients that you may have overlooked.

EQUIPMENT FOR WORKING IN THE HOME

Spoon Measurement Get an excellent set of stainless steel ones. They will last a long time. They'll serve you well for a long time to come.

Cups for Measuring Dry measuring cups are used for all of the measures in this recipe book. Most of these are made of metal and have a flat handle, making them unrecognisable as belonging to your grandma. Affirmed that this will be your method? Great! Everyone, get ready for the next tool.

Spatulas for icing These tools are used in a few recipes that need the application of frosting and glaze. If you don't have a professional-looking knife, this one does the trick.

Brush for basting I'm not afraid to use my fists. Making tins greased with paper towels is wasteful, and drizzling with oil is difficult. To accomplish these duties, a basting brush comes in handy. Brushing pastries is also a great use for it.

The rolling pin It doesn't matter. The type without handles is the one I like. An empty wine bottle will do in a pinch.

Melon Baller/Ice Cream Scoop Melons are great for making cookies because they're easy to handle and don't leave your hands covered in goop. For cookies, I use a 1-inch melon-baller, but you may use whatever size you prefer—just keep an eye on the cooking times.

Squeeze Bottle Made of Plastic In order to drizzle Wonder Buns and other items with sauce, this is required.

Gingerbread men and sugar cookies can be made with this cookie cutter. It's up to you which forms you choose to purchase, although you should definitely go crazy and acquire any that even pique your curiosity.

Oven Temperature Probe This is strictly for the purpose of preventing potential harm. If you want to keep your skin young, grab one of these and keep an eye on it!

CULINARY UTILITIES

Trays Shaped in a Unique Way Makeleine pans and heart-shaped pans are required to make several of the recipes in this book, in addition to the standard baking sheet.

The pans used to make donuts This type is widely available, although you may or may not enjoy it according to its chemical composition. The same is true for me, but I'm glad to announce that I'm doing my best to remedy the situation now. The BabyCakes website is updated frequently, so be sure to check back.

Pans for bread (7 x 4 x 3). If you happen to have a smaller one sitting around, feel free to use it. It's critical, though, that you don't overfill your pan. Make muffins with the extra batter.

Embossed Parchment If you don't line the pans with parchment paper, baked items will stick to them. Wax paper is a poor replacement; do not use it.

Cake Rounds/Baking Sheets Baking sheets that promise ideal cookie baking aren't worth the extra money, in my opinion. It's best to use parchment paper to line any old rimmed baking sheet or cookie tray for these recipes.

A Waffle Maker Do you have a family? Do you have any acquaintances who have tied the knot? A waffle iron was presumably given to you or given to you as a gift if you said yes to either question. It's time to bring it back to life. In the absence of one, go to the nearest mall and get the cheapest option; there is no way around the fact that they are all untidy.

This book is completely gluten-free—nothing in it contains it.

Because this is why.

When I sat down to brainstorm the contents of this book, I was confronted with a number of difficult choices. One of the most pressing is whether or not I should continue to include spelt-based baked goods in this book, as I did in the first? Spelt is a relative of wheat that many wheat-intolerant people, including myself, can eat without difficulty. In the gluten-free vs. spelt bread war, the numbers are roughly equal based on a blind bakery count. Every time a gluten-free product is sold, a spelt-based one is also purchased. What a quandary! I couldn't help but ponder.

The spelt loyalist faction made it clear that they were relying on this book's recipes for Wonder Buns, Honey Buns, and Hamentaschen, all of which are traditionally baked with spelt. I couldn't leave them out. Not a day goes by that we don't receive an urgent call from a customer pleading with us to help them convert the spelt recipe in the first book to one that is gluten-free. That's when it became evident that I needed to get back into the kitchen and squirm my way toward a gluten-free, vegan, agave sweetened pastry dough. Problem was, no matter how many times I tried, I was unable to come up with an appropriate and delicious gluten-free pastry crust to go with any of my previous recipes. It was like trying to solve a huge Rubik's Cube of ingredients, and I was never going to be able to.

However, I enjoy a good challenge, so I jumped right in, feeling re-energized and ready to go. My usual errors resulted in the creation of an unfathomably grody dough. I was so close to giving up, my lord! That is when I realised how beautiful my victories over these ingredients had been in the past, so I kept going. I reduced the amount of flour, increased the amount of arrowroot, and increased the amount of vanilla until I had the right crust that was mild, delicate, and sweet, yet strong enough to hold up to the squishy fillings.

So that I could replicate the classic Sanka advertising, I put the finished Wonder Bun through its paces with Skinny Bun consumers who had already had their spelt cleared. The look on gluten-intolerant regulars' faces as they hoarded them by the bagful was reward enough for everyone's amazement. As a result of the event, I'm now a 100-year-old man.

BabyCakes NYC's gluten-free recipe book. There is a new path ahead...

As an added bonus for Spelt Lovers, I've included in The Rules of Substitutions a conversion chart for gluten-free to spelt flour. (It's all good!)

Chapter Two

HOW DO I KNOW WHERE TO GET STARTED?

This is an excellent query. The new Piece of Cake rating system can be seen next to each recipe title in this book. Everything you've ever wanted to know can be found here. There are four coloured slices of cake lined up neatly in a row to illustrate how difficult a dish is compared to the rest of the book in this system. There are four levels of difficulty: one, two, three, and four. As an illustration, consider the following recipe rating:

According to the BabyCakes NYC Piece of Cake grading scale, the preceding recipe merits a three-piece cake. Please, use this as a reference point. Those of you who are knowledgeable with your money will benefit greatly from my advice. Choose simple recipes while you're just getting started so you don't squander any valuable ingredients. The Wonder Buns and other similarly advanced dishes are perfect for anyone on the cusp of professional status. There's always opportunity for improvement here.

What questions do you have? We have answers.

I'm always up for a good challenge. As a self-confessed question-asker, I have high regard for persons who appreciate the value of pestering those who are more knowledgeable than they are. The fact that I still work the floor and ovens at each BabyCakes NYC location means that I have a unique perspective on what you're thinking about even before you realise it. As a teaser, here's what I'

That's terrible. Oh my God! My recipe yielded more batter than I expected, so now what? Why?

At the bakery, we've all been there. Even when we believe we are following the recipe to the letter, we end up with too much batter. In other words, here's the deal: When it comes to measurements, they sometimes have their own minds of their own. In this case, it's possible that the flour in your bag was packed too tightly, causing an overabundance in the measuring dish. Other times, it's because the baker accidentally overmeasured the oil, agave, or applesauce. Your recipe is in danger at this time. Are you short on time? First, you may want to bake the remaining batter and see how it turns out, if you're able. As long as you're comfortable with your ingredients, all you have to do is tweak the entire batch and you're good to go!

The nut milk craze continues unabated. Can I use those in place of the rice milk you recommended?

The sky is the limit as long as you're willing to take a risk and fail at least twice before giving up. Although I haven't tested substituting nut milks for rice milk, I'm convinced in their efficacy.

This is what my cookies look like after they were run over by a station waggon. What's the deal with that?

Perhaps you over-measured the oil or under-measured the flour in your recipe. If you like your cookies more cake-like, you can add 14 cup more flour the next time you make them.

Please note that the potato flour in my pantry is not potato starch, although I do have a little of it on hand if that helps. Is that anything you'd recommend using?

Nope! It has to be potato starch. Never ever use potato flour. Potato flour, on the other hand, I have no idea what it's used for.

The flour made from garbanzo beans is an option. Are garbanzo bean flour and fava bean flour interchangeable?

Sorry! For this recipe, the only bean flours acceptable are garbanzo and fava bean.

When I put my baked good in the oven, it came out all goopy, even though I followed the recipe to the letter. That's a tough one.

This is a difficult one. All ovens aren't created equal. When we launched our bakery in Los Angeles, I was forced to learn this painful lesson. I acquired the same same oven that we use in our New York flagship, but I realised that the new one took more time with the recipes — presumably growing pains — than the old one. After the halfway point, check your baked item every five minutes and remove it from the oven when the middle is cooked through.

It's going to be melted! If the temperature of the coconut oil dips below 66 degrees, it will solidify, so reheat it for about 25 seconds in the microwave or in a skillet on low heat before using it in the measuring cup.

Coconut dominates the flavour profile of all of my baked items. There is nothing I can do about it.

Omega Nutrition 100 Percent Organic Coconut Oil is odourless at BabyCakes NYC. When correctly handled, this product has a butter-like texture that is almost indescribable.

Coconut oil, oh my, is incredibly fattening. Please provide more details.

Coconut oil is an extremely misunderstood food. But not all saturated fats are the same; this one is. There are no trans-fatty acids in it. Lauric acid, an important fatty acid, is abundant in this oil. Those who are immune-suppressed may benefit from the antiviral effects of lauric acid, which is also found in breast milk, where it helps prevent the spread of bacteria and viruses. Use coconut oil against your apprehensions if you must, and see what happens.

I've come to the conclusion that coconut oil is not for me. Is it possible to substitute a different type of oil for this one?

Yes, that's correct. Other scentless oils such as rice bran oil and grapeseed are excellent substitutes for canola oil if canola doesn't work for you. It's only when you're making the BabyCakes NYC icing and frosting that things go wrong. Coconut oil is required for this recipe; any other oil will result in an unsatisfactory result.

Agave nectar: light or dark?

Organic Nectars' light agave is my preference, and I'll tell you why: Dark agave is simply too powerful. My recipes do include it, at least. The lighter version brings out the flavours of the other ingredients and unifies the dish as a whole.

CONVENTIONS RELATING TO SUBSTITUTION

It appears that many of you have items you'd like to avoid and others you'd like to add, so I've included this list of alternatives. So that's good to know. To be honest, I hope I could compose a recipe that would satisfy everyone's cravings every time, but I doubt I'll be able to do so before I'm a very old person. Listed below are some guidelines I use while I'm experimenting with new ways to create recipes. They are not impenetrable by any means, however.

Adapting Gluten-Free Recipes for Spelt

Spelt is a grain that we utilise at the BabyCakes NYC locations (all materials and tools for spelt recipes are carefully kept separate from the gluten-free ones, believe me) despite the fact that I didn't use it in this collection of recipes. In spite of this, I'm sure some people will refuse to use it because of their sensitivity to gluten. People who aren't allergic to gluten may prefer the fluffier, softer crumb of spelt over the thick, muffin-like texture of gluten-free bread. This means you can adapt one of my gluten-free recipes (and save some money on supplies) by substituting spelt flour for wheat flour. Sum up your gluten free flour, potato starch and arrowroot measures before substituting spelt flour in place of them all at once. Instead of 2 cups of gluten-free flour, 14 cup of potato starch, and 14 cup of arrowroot, use 2 12 cups of spelt flour in the same recipe. Xanthan gum and water should be omitted due to the spelt flour's unique qualities (if the recipe calls for it). Everything is taken care of for you by using spelt flour.

RECIPE TRANSFORMATION FROM VEGAN SUGARS TO AGAVE-SWEETENED RECIPE

Cookies and brownies can have a crispy, chewy texture thanks to the use of unrefined vegan sugar, such Florida Crystals. For each cup of vegan sugar you replace with agave nectar, you can substitute 23 cup of agave nectar. Here's a cautionary tale: Reduce your total wet components by 13 cup because of the liquid nature of agave nectar.

In most circumstances, the oil will be the primary component. Rice milk or fruit puree may be used in some circumstances. A teaspoon-by-teaspoon reduction of a mixture of substances may also be necessary in some situations. This is your experiment, and you're sailing in hazardous waters that I normally avoid..... My best piece of advice is to be patient and discover what works best over time. Remember to take notes! If something works, make a note of it so you don't have to worry about converting it again. The only thing I can say for sure is that the texture will change from crunchy to spongy and cake-like.

EXCLUSIVELY for those who do not want to use either vegan sugar or Agave in their recipes.

Using coconut sugar instead of vegan sugar is a no-brainer for me because I'm a huge fan of coconut. Because coconut sugar is so hard to come by and so expensive, I decided not to include it in this cookbook. It's worth it for some dishes, but I think you'll agree that it's a bit excessive. If you do decide to give it a go, simply use 1 cup of coconut sugar for every 2 and a half cups of agave nectar instead of the vegan sugar. It's important to keep in mind that I haven't tried coconut sugar in every recipe. The recipes, on the other hand, won't be as chewy and they'll have a stronger caramel taste.

A SUBSTITUTE FOR BEAN FLOUR, IF YOU PREFER.

Garbanzo and fava bean flour or Bob's Red Mill All-Purpose Gluten-Free Baking Flour are two of my favourite gluten-free flour substitutes since they make cakes and muffins far more fluffy than rice flour. It is possible to substitute rice flour in place of the garbanzo and fava bean mixture if you are allergic to beans. A mixture of 2 cups rice flour, 34 cup potato starch, and 1 cup arrowroot, mixed together, seems to work well in recipes that call for Bob's Red Mill All-Purpose Gluten-Free Baking Flour substitutes. (3 cups plus 1 tablespoon of flour are produced.)

RECIPE FOR BREAKFAST

MOST OF US HAVE SOME KIND OF FREAKY DAILY BUGABOO that starts the moment the first ray of sunlight hits our face.

Me? While cutting a grapefruit into a dozen pieces in the dark with one eye closed, I stagger into the kitchen, prepare tea, and moan about not going to the gym. Every day at 5:30 a.m., and grapefruit does not count as breakfast.

When I walk into the bakery and see the array of still-warm muffins, biscuits, scones, and tea cakes that the first shift of bakers has produced, it's magic time. It's a Neverland that everyone shares. But, until recently, I had always despised those leisurely sit-down pancake and waffle breakfasts. That luxury vanished around the time I was in my late teens. My mother is to blame for allowing me to leave the house in the first place. Welcome to the chapter that puts things right for those who share this nostalgia.

My recipes for a range of breakfast staples that are suitable for vegans, celiacs, and gluten-free eaters can be found here. That's right, we're tackling three titans, as well as a few variants on them: pancakes (oh!), waffles (gasp!), and cinnamon buns (yes!). Did I remember to include maple syrup? Yes! Before you start, you should definitely get someone to arrange the table so you don't have to wait long to plate.

Chapter Three

PANCAKES

Pancakes! Apart from ice cream, pancakes are without a doubt my favourite food. Is it surprising that a gluten- and dairy-free baker would say that? Probably. In any case, here's the recipe, complete with all the buttery pleasure. Please keep in mind that I prefer my pancakes very thin, so expect that from this recipe. Simply add another 13 cup flour to make them meatier.

Do you want another no-brainer dish to accompany this one? How about a somewhat billowy core with a sweet aftertaste and mildly chunky texture of banana mashed up against the crispy outlines of the pancake crust? Already, take the day off! Personally, I sometimes add pre-mashed bananas to produce a delicate fruit-to-batter mélange, and by that I mean in this recipe. However, if you're a breakfast bungee-jumper or something, you could rough them up and make a deliciously rocky stack.

2 cups Bob's Red Mill Gluten-Free All-Purpose Baking Flour

2 teaspoons bicarbonate of soda

2 tblsp. baking powder

1 teaspoon cinnamon powder

1 tblsp. salt

xanthan gum (12 teaspoon)

agave nectar (23 cup)

2/3 gallon rice milk

2/3 cup applesauce, unsweetened

12 cup melted refined coconut or canola oil, plus a little extra for the pan

2 tbsp vanilla essence

Maple Agave Syrup

PANCAKES WITH BANANAS

2/3 cup mashed or diced banana

Combine the flour, baking soda, baking powder, cinnamon, salt, and xanthan gum in a medium mixing bowl. With a rubber spatula, combine the agave nectar, rice milk, applesauce, 12 cup coconut oil, and vanilla until the batter is smooth. If used, mix in the banana.

Over medium heat, heat a large nonstick skillet or pancake griddle. 1 teaspoon coconut oil, tilted back and forth in the pan to coat it Pour 14-cup amounts of the batter into the pan in batches. Cook for 3 minutes, or until the batter is dimpled with tiny holes on the majority of the surface, then flip. Cook for another 2 minutes on the other side, or until the middle of the pancake bounces back when tapped and it is golden brown. Repeat with the remaining batter and place the pancakes on a heated plate. Serve with Agave Maple Syrup on the side.

12–14 servings

PANCAKES WITH GINGERBREAD

What could be a better wintertime breakfast than this? The nicest aspect about this recipe, in my opinion, is that it fulfils all of your gingerbread fancies in a quick and easy way that avoids the hassle of making a full gingerbread loaf. I'll admit it now, sheepishly: I've been known to forego the maple syrup and instead smother these in vanilla frosting or glaze... for breakfast. Please, before you pass judgement, give me the benefit of the doubt and try it for yourself.

2 cups Bob's Red Mill Gluten-Free All-Purpose Baking Flour

2 teaspoons bicarbonate of soda

2 tblsp. baking powder

1 tablespoon ginger powder

1 teaspoon cinnamon powder

1 tblsp. salt

xanthan gum (12 teaspoon)

14 teaspoon cardamom powder

14 teaspoon clove powder

2/3 cup applesauce, unsweetened

12 cup melted refined coconut or canola oil, plus a little extra for the pan

agave nectar (13 cup)

13 cup molasses (dark)

2/3 gallon rice milk

2 tbsp vanilla essence

Maple Agave Syrup

Combine the flour, baking soda, baking powder, ginger, cinnamon, salt, xanthan gum, cardamom, and cloves in a medium mixing bowl. With a rubber spatula, stir in the applesauce, 12 cup coconut oil, agave nectar, molasses, rice milk, and vanilla until the batter is smooth.

1 teaspoon coconut oil, heated in a large nonstick skillet or on a griddle over medium heat. Pour 14 cup pancake batter into the pan for each pancake, working in batches. Spread the batter with the back of a rubber spatula to produce a 4-inch pancake. Cook for 2 minutes on one side, then turn and cook for another 2 minutes on the other side, or until the centre bounces back and the edges are golden. Repeat with the remaining batter and place the pancakes on a heated plate. Serve with Agave Maple Syrup on the side.

12–14 servings

Chapter Four

BUNS OF WONDER

Even the faintest aroma of cinnamon and melted sugar is enough to transport any lady back to her childhood food court. When we make a batch of this dish, it takes centre stage at the bakery, which is no small feat given the competition of fragrant apple muffins, rich cornbread, and dozens of other aromatic samples. BabyCakes NYC's Wonder Buns offer everything you've been looking for: a delicately sticky chewiness, spicy pockets mixed in with sweet streaks of delight, and a dense but layered structure that's the stuff of dreams.

GLUTEN-FREE BASIC PASTRY DOUGH

114 cup Bob's Red Mill Gluten-Free All-Purpose Baking Flour

12 cup rice flour (brown)

14 cup arrowroot powder

xanthan gum (134 teaspoons)

1 tablespoon powdered sugar

1 tablespoon cinnamon powder

14 cup refined coconut or canola oil, melted

agave nectar (13 cup)

3 tbsp vanilla essence

1 cup of hot water

rice flour (12 cup)

14 cup refined coconut or canola oil, melted

agave nectar (12 cup)

3 teaspoons cinnamon powder

12 c. raisins (optional)

4 tablespoons icing sugar

Preheat the oven to 325 degrees Fahrenheit. Set aside 2 rimmed baking sheets lined with parchment paper.

Whisk together the gluten-free all-purpose flour, 12 cup rice flour, arrowroot, xanthan gum, baking powder, and 1 tablespoon cinnamon in a medium mixing basin. With a rubber spatula, whisk in 14 cup coconut oil, 13 cup agave nectar, and the vanilla until a very thick dry dough forms. Add a third of a cup of warm water at a time until the dough is slightly sticky, stirring in more as needed. Refrigerate for 20 minutes after wrapping in plastic.

Turn the dough out onto a surface coated with 13 cup rice flour in the centre. Roll out the dough into a 12-inch-thick rectangle with the short side facing you, dusting the top of the dough and a rolling pin with some of the leftover rice flour. Apply half of the remaining coconut oil to the dough's surface with a pastry brush.

12 cup agave nectar and 3 teaspoons cinnamon, combined in a small bowl. Brush the mixture over the dough, completely coating it. Evenly distribute the raisins throughout the mixture.

Begin rolling the dough into a log, starting with the short side closest to you. To produce 12 rolls, cut the log into 1-inch-wide pieces using a very sharp knife. Place 6 rolls on each of the baking pans that have been prepped. Remove from the oven after 12 minutes and brush the tops and edges of each bun with the remaining coconut oil. Bake for an additional 5 minutes, or until the sides are golden brown and the centres are somewhat soft. Allow it cool for 10 minutes before serving with a teaspoon of Vanilla Icing on each bun.

12 servings

BUNS OF HONEY

Honey is on the "absolutely not, you jerk" list for the majority of vegans. And that's all right. But what should one do in such circumstances? Naturally, I reach for my not-so-secret weapon, agave nectar. EZ-PZ! The Honey Buns recipe is essentially a tweaked Wonder Bun recipe that has been infused with honey and topped with vegan sugar for texture. The extra sweetness from the honey-agave makes for a great day-starter when you don't want to listen to your alarm clock.

1 cup sugar (vegan)

4 teaspoons cinnamon powder

34 cup refined coconut or canola oil, melted

14 cup agave nectar plus 13 cup

114 cup Bob's Red Mill Gluten-Free All-Purpose Baking Flour

12 cup brown rice flour plus an additional 12 cup for dusting

14 cup arrowroot powder

1 tablespoon powdered sugar

xanthan gum (134 teaspoons)

3 tbsp vanilla essence

34 cup hot water

Preheat the oven to 325 degrees Fahrenheit. Set aside 2 rimmed baking sheets lined with parchment paper.

Whisk together the sugar and 3 tablespoons of cinnamon in a small bowl and set aside. In a separate small dish, combine 14 cup coconut oil and 14 cup agave nectar and leave aside.

Whisk together the all-purpose gluten-free flour, 12 cup rice flour, arrowroot, baking powder, remaining 1 tablespoon cinnamon, and xanthan gum in a medium mixing basin. With a rubber spatula, whisk in 14 cup coconut oil, 13 cup agave nectar, and the vanilla until a very thick dry dough forms. Add the warm water gradually until the dough is somewhat sticky. Refrigerate for 20 minutes after wrapping in plastic.

Turn the dough out onto a surface coated with 13 cup rice flour in the centre. Roll out the dough into a 12-inch-thick rectangle with the short side facing you, dusting the top of the dough and a rolling pin with the remaining rice flour.

Apply a thick coat of coconut oil to the dough's surface with a pastry brush. Half of the cinnamon-sugar mixture should be sprinkled over the dough, completely coating it.

Begin rolling the dough into a log, starting with the short side closest to you. To produce 12 rolls, cut the log into 1-inch-wide pieces using a very sharp knife. Place 6 rolls on each of the baking pans that have been prepped. Brush half of the coconut oil–agave nectar mixture onto each bun, then top with the remaining cinnamon-sugar mixture.

Remove the buns from the oven after 12 minutes and brush the tops and sides with the leftover coconut oil–agave nectar mixture. Bake for a further 10 minutes, or until the edges are golden brown and the middle is somewhat soft. Remove the dish from the oven and set it aside to cool for 10 minutes before serving.

12 servings

LET'S GET STARTED

After the hundredth time making Honey Buns and Wonder Buns, you'll look at your pastry dough and think, "You know, pastry dough, I bet there's something else I can do to you." This is something I wholeheartedly support. My contributions to your efforts are listed here.

Roll of Jelly Replace the agave, cinnamon, and raisin mixture in the Wonder Buns with 34 cup of your favourite jam, which you should spread over the dough before rolling it. Here are my favourite jam flavours for this, in descending order: strawberry, raspberry, and blackberry

Chocolate Cake What exactly are you saying? Is this Madeleine's charmingly insubordinate cousin-in-law? Yep! The Honey Bun recipe works best for the BabyCakes NYC pain au chocolat: All you have to do is generously sprinkle 2/3 cup chocolate chips over the surface of the pastry dough before rolling it up. Sprinkle a little vegan sugar on top of your dough and bake as usual.

Twists of Cinnamon This one is a little more difficult, but don't be alarmed. Cut the Wonder Bun pastry dough into as many equal-width strips as you'd like (I generally go for 24). Pinch the ends of your pieces as you twist and/or braid them together. Bake till golden brown, then sprinkle with cinnamon and vegan sugar. Put your kids to work on this one if you have them.

Chapter Five

WAFFLES

There are few things I love more than the mix of salty and sweet, from cornbread covered with jam to peanut butter and jelly. After figuring out the pancake recipe, it occurred to me—thanks to an Eggo-heavy childhood—that a waffle recipe would be the ideal way to delve deeper into the salty-sweet relationship. A dab of coconut oil and a pinch of salt on each waffle before adding the Agave Maple Syrup is ideal for me.

Is there anything better? Making chocolate-chip cookies! If you chance to come across that beautiful department loaded with every known variation of organic, sweetened, unsweetened, and flavoured chocolate while wandering the grocery store aisles, make sure to tackle it full force. Then rush over to the vegan whipped cream and grab some. Put some vegan powdered sugar in your shopping cart. Get on the phone and offer up your waffle-making services to anyone willing to clean up the mess you're about to make by loading these groceries into your trunk or into your small go-cart to push home.

14 cup melted refined coconut or canola oil, plus a little extra to grease the waffle iron (or use gluten-free, vegan nonstick spray)

12 cup Bob's Red Mill Gluten-Free All-Purpose Baking Flour

1 cup rice flour (brown)

2 tblsp. baking powder

1 teaspoon bicarbonate of soda

1 tblsp. salt

xanthan gum (34 teaspoon)

rice milk (212 cup)

agave nectar (3 tablespoons)

1 teaspoon of vanilla extract

Maple Agave Syrup

WAFFLES WITH CHOCOLATE CHIP

1 cup gluten-free vegan chocolate chips

12 cup powdered vegan sugar for sprinkling

Preheat a waffle maker as directed by the manufacturer. Spray the iron with gluten-free, vegan nonstick spray or brush it with oil.

Whisk together the flours, baking powder, baking soda, salt, and xanthan gum in a medium mixing basin. With a rubber spatula, blend the rice milk, 14 cup coconut oil, agave nectar, and vanilla (plus chocolate chips, if preferred).

Pour 13 to 12 cup batter onto the waffle griddle and bake until done to your liking (or as directed by the manufacturer). Remove the waffle from the griddle and top with Agave Maple Syrup to serve (and with a dusting of powdered sugar for chocolate-chip waffles). Rep with the rest of the batter.

It serves 12 people.

SYRUP OF AGAVE MAPLE

Pay attention: Maple syrup is high in manganese and zinc (both beneficial minerals), yet it is still one of the world's most delectable sweeteners. Unfortunately, the stuff's high sugar level will send me to the hospital if I look at it for too long. Can you guess what I did to compensate without looking at the recipe name again? Did you just say the word agave under your breath? You and I, I believe we're finally getting somewhere. I laboured extensively on producing this substitute maple elixir I promise you'll enjoy in between hours spent tweaking and perfecting the pancake and waffle recipes.

1 agave nectar cup

3 tbsp maple flavouring (or to taste)

In a small bowl, pour the agave nectar. Stir in the maple flavour until it is completely blended. Taste and adjust the maple flavour to your liking. The syrup can be kept at room temperature for up to a month if firmly covered.

Approximately 1 cup

Chapter Six

CREPES

CREPE WITH CARAMELIZED ONION AND CHEDDAR CHEESE

Do you have a habit of grabbing whatever savoury dinner leftovers are in the refrigerator the next morning? Or perhaps you're the type who is just as likely to throw together a quick salad as you are to gobble a donut as soon as you get out of bed. What do you think? Do you like pancakes for dinner? I understand and sympathise with you. What I eat and when I eat it has no real rhyme or reason, and some mornings I just can't bear the thought of an indulgent treat, no matter how perfectly prepared it is. To that goal, we must restore the savoury breakfast's gluten-free status. As a result, I made some crepes. These guys are ridiculously simple to make, and you'll have a hot, cheese-dripping supper in front of you in less than fifteen minutes. Plus, don't they have a nice ring to them? If you don't have time to caramelise the onion, these are still delicious.

CREPE

34 cup Bob's Red Mill Gluten-Free All-Purpose Baking Flour

14 cup rice flour (brown)

xanthan gum (12 teaspoon)

14 teaspoon kosher salt

14 cup heated refined coconut or canola oil, plus a little extra for coating the pan

12 gallon rice milk

34 cup boiling water

FILLING

2 tbsp refined coconut oil, canola oil, or olive oil, melted

1 cup yellow onion, chopped

12 teaspoon salt + a little extra for sprinkling

12 teaspoon black pepper, plus salt and pepper to taste

1 vegan cheddar cheese cup

To prepare the crepes, whisk together the flours, xanthan gum, and salt in a medium mixing bowl. With a rubber spatula, whisk in the coconut oil, rice milk, and boiling water until a thin batter forms.

Over medium-high heat, heat a low-sided 8-inch skillet or crepe pan. Brush the bottom of the skillet with the remaining 18 tsp coconut oil. Fill the pan with 13 cup batter and rotate it to coat the entire surface. Cook the crepe for 1 minute or until the top is dry. Flip the crepe with the spatula below it. Cook for another minute or until golden, then transfer to a cooling rack or dish. Rep with the rest of the batter.

To create the filling, melt 1 tablespoon coconut oil in a large sauté pan. Cook, stirring occasionally, until the onion is tender and nearly transparent, about 4 minutes. Cook until the cheese has melted, adding salt and pepper as needed.

Place the crepe on a work area and cover it with a layer of filling. Close the crepe and season with a pinch of salt. Carry on until all of the crepes have been dressed. Serve right away.

12 servings

Chapter Seven

TART WITH VEGETABLES

So one fateful Sunday morning, you invited everyone around for brunch. Sunday! You sleep until eleven o'clock, don't wash your hair or change out of your pyjamas, and end up watching TV upside down on the couch with newspapers and gossip magazines strewn about the floor. Tsk-tsk, it doesn't appear that you're quite ready for the hostess habit you picked up along the way. Nonetheless, here we are! Thank goodness for this brunch-ready recipe that you can make the night before without even your most obnoxious gourmet buddies noticing. Simply prepare your dough and vegetables and refrigerate them overnight in the refrigerator. Simply follow the baking directions in the morning. If you don't like sweet potatoes, try substituting 34 cup sautéed mushrooms.

CRUST

114 cup Bob's Red Mill Gluten-Free All-Purpose Baking Flour

12 cup brown rice flour plus an additional 12 cup for dusting

14 cup arrowroot powder

1 tablespoon powdered sugar

salt (2 tablespoons)

xanthan gum, 112 tablespoons

14 cup melted refined coconut or canola oil, with a little extra for brushing the dough

agave nectar (2 teaspoons)

1 cup of hot water

FILLING

12 cup refined coconut or canola oil, melted

1 small sweet potato, 12 inch thickly sliced

Salt

12 cup leeks, thinly sliced

1 medium zucchini, thinly sliced

1 thinly sliced medium red bell pepper

3 minced garlic cloves

rosemary, 1 teaspoon (fresh or dried)

12 tsp. chilli flakes (optional)

12 cup vegan gluten-free grated cheese

Using parchment paper, line the bottom of a 9-inch-round tart pan (you do not need to line the sides).

To prepare the crust, whisk together the flours, arrowroot, baking powder, salt, and xanthan gum in a medium mixing bowl. Using a rubber spatula, continue mixing in the coconut oil and agave nectar.

Slowly drizzle in the water until a thick dough forms. Refrigerate the dough for 20 minutes after wrapping it in plastic. Turn the dough out onto a work surface coated with 13 cup rice flour in the centre. Roll out the dough into a 14-inch-thick rectangle, dusting the top of the dough and a rolling pin with the remaining rice flour.

Allow the excess dough to fall over the edges as you transfer the rolled-out pastry dough to the prepared tart pan. Cut away any excess dough with a knife and discard. Set aside after pressing the dough into the pan and brushing it with coconut oil.

Preheat the oven to 375°F for the filling. Set aside a rimmed baking sheet lined with parchment paper and brushed with coconut oil.

Brush the sweet potato slices with coconut oil, season with salt, and bake for 20 minutes, or until they are soft. Place aside.

In a large skillet, melt 2 tablespoons coconut oil over medium heat. Sauté for 8 minutes with the leeks, zucchini, and bell pepper. Cook for a further 4 minutes, or until the veggies are tender, adding the garlic, rosemary, 1 teaspoon salt, and chilli flakes, if using.

Place the sweet potato on top of the crust, then equally distribute the veggie mixture. Cheese should be sprinkled on top. Bake for 25 minutes, until the cheese has melted and the crust has turned golden brown.

Approximately 8 slices

Chapter Eight

GRANOLA

Every morning, not everyone has time to sit down to a dish of freshly prepared waffles or crepes. Before you wonder who would want to undertake such a thing, let me state unequivocally that I would. However, I understand what you're saying. Granola is a great substitute for a traditional sit-down breakfast—a it's naturally light and simple option that's just as filling as any other baked breakfast item. When I travel, I keep this in a small baggie so I don't go hungry when the flight attendants pass by selling sodium-soaked chips or dried-up cookies.

4 cups oats (gluten-free)

1 tblsp. salt

1 tablespoon cinnamon powder

1 teaspoon ginger powder

12 cup coconut (unsweetened)

pecans, 1 cup (optional)

1 cup berries, dried (I prefer blueberries and cranberries)

13 cup refined coconut or canola oil, melted

agave nectar (13 cup)

Preheat the oven to 350 degrees Fahrenheit. Set aside a rimmed baking sheet lined with parchment paper.

Mix together the oats, salt, cinnamon, ginger, coconut, pecans (if using), and dried berries in a medium bowl. Toss in the coconut oil and agave nectar until the oats are completely covered. Pour the mixture onto the baking sheet that has been prepared. Bake for 15 minutes, then toss and bake for an additional 10 to 15 minutes, or until golden brown. Remove the granola from the oven and set aside to cool completely before serving.

12 people

RECIPES FOR COOKIES

With all the baking, book writing, and hair appointments, I haven't travelled the globe much, but one thing is certain: cookies make the world go 'round. The challenge in compiling a list of some of my favourite iconic cookies for this book was determining which ones had to be included. The outcome is the longest chapter in the book.

Now I realise I've forgotten some perennial favourites. Many of you will be disappointed that there isn't a gluten-free Nutter Butter or a vegan-friendly Double Stuf. To you, I say, "Perhaps next time." I'll add this for you: It's no exaggeration to say that the eleven brand-new recipes I created for this part will help you entirely reinvent what is possible in the cookie sphere for vegans, celiacs, gluten-free people, and health-conscious people. What do you mean, Thin Mints? Madeleines? Snickerdoodles?

Furthermore, many of these recipes—like my silent hero, the sugar cookie—allow you to explore and add new and unusual tastes to fit your preferences. However, you'll need to stick close by my side in a few other spots; things may get a little complicated at times, and some of these cookies are really finicky. In every situation, I tell you, it is well worth the effort.

Chapter Nine

MINTS THIN

I was raised Catholic. To us, winter signifies Lent, which, aside from school clothes, is about all I remember. When winter/Lent arrived, the only thing we could bank on was an increase in house-wide hatred as we avoided sweets and desserts in all their overindulgent forms for several weeks. Girl Scout cookie season, as you may recall, is during the winter months. Rather than simply not ordering from the Scouts, our family ordered a few, placed them in the freezer, and froze them until Easter, which was about two months later. This recipe is for all those gluten-free people who have never been able to enjoy a winter of Girl Scout Thin Mints—and for all you weak-willed kids who can't stop themselves from breaking the Lenten fast. Your hearts are blessed!

12 cup Bob's Red Mill Gluten-Free All-Purpose Baking Flour

1 cup sugar (vegan)

12 cup cocoa powder, unsweetened

14 cup arrowroot powder

xanthan gum, 112 tablespoons

1 teaspoon bicarbonate of soda

1 tblsp. salt

34 cup refined coconut or canola oil, melted

13 cup applesauce, unsweetened

2 tbsp vanilla essence

1 cup gluten-free vegan chocolate chips

3 tablespoons extract de mint

Preheat the oven to 325 degrees Fahrenheit. Set aside 2 rimmed baking sheets lined with parchment paper.

Whisk together the flour, sugar, cocoa powder, arrowroot, xanthan gum, baking soda, and salt in a medium mixing basin. With a rubber spatula, combine the coconut oil, applesauce, and vanilla until a thick dough forms.

Using a teaspoon, drop the dough onto the prepared baking sheets, spacing them 112 inches apart. Flatten each dough mound gently with your fingertips, flattening the edges. Bake for 7 minutes, then rotate the baking sheets and continue baking for another 7 minutes. Allow 15 minutes to cool on the baking sheets.

Meanwhile, in a small saucepan over medium heat, combine the chocolate chips and mint essence. Stir constantly until the chips are completely melted. Avoid overcooking. Turn off the heat. Dip the tops of each cookie in the melted chocolate and arrange them on a dish in a single layer. Refrigerate for 30 minutes, or until the chocolate has hardened.

30 servings

Chapter Ten

AHOY, CHIPS!

I'm a lady who enjoys her cookies thin, chewy, and buttery to the point of obsession. I go to the cake department when I want a piece of cake. This isn't to suggest that the gigantic and fairly hefty Chips Ahoy! was not the preeminent cookie of my youth. And certainly not those M&M-flecked late-issue monsters. I'm talking about the authentic original flavour, all dry and crumbly. This is my take on the delightfully titled cookie.

oat flour 112 cup

1 cup Bob's Red Mill Gluten-Free All-Purpose Baking Flour

1 cup sugar (vegan)

14 cup flaxseed meal

14 cup arrowroot powder

xanthan gum, 112 tablespoons

1 teaspoon bicarbonate of soda

1 tblsp. salt

heated refined coconut oil or canola oil (34 cup plus 2 teaspoons)

6 tbsp. applesauce, unsweetened

2 tbsp vanilla essence

1 cup gluten-free vegan chocolate chips

Preheat the oven to 325 degrees Fahrenheit. Set aside 2 rimmed baking sheets lined with parchment paper.

Whisk together the flours, sugar, flax meal, arrowroot, xanthan gum, baking soda, and salt in a medium mixing bowl. With a rubber spatula, whisk in the coconut oil, applesauce, and vanilla until a thick dough forms. Add the chocolate chunks and stir until they are uniformly distributed.

Drop the dough onto the prepared baking sheets by the teaspoonful, about 112 inches apart. Bake for 7 minutes, then move the baking sheets and bake for an additional 7 minutes, or until golden brown and firm. Allow for 15 minutes on the baking sheets before serving.

COOKIES IN BLACK-AND-WHITE

For a long time, I thought I was the only person in the tristate area who had never heard of the gorgeous enormous black-and-white cookies that could be found in every bodega from Brooklyn to the Bronx. Have you ever tried one? Of course, because of my food sensitivity, I was never allowed. So when I walked into the kitchen to come up with cookie ideas, this was one of the first that sprang to me. Prepare to be surrounded by the delicious warmth of vanilla-chocolate overabundance.

114 cup rice flour (white or brown)

12 cup Bob's Red Mill Gluten-Free All-Purpose Baking Flour

13 cup sugar (vegan)

12 cup arrowroot powder

xanthan gum, 112 tablespoons

1 teaspoon bicarbonate of soda

1 tblsp. salt

34 cup refined coconut or canola oil, melted

13 cup unsweetened applesauce plus 2 teaspoons

agave nectar (13 cup)

2 tbsp vanilla essence

Glaze with Vanilla Sugar

Chocolate Dipping Sauce with Sugar

Preheat the oven to 325 degrees Fahrenheit. Set aside 2 rimmed baking sheets lined with parchment paper.

Whisk together the flours, sugar, arrowroot, xanthan gum, baking soda, and salt in a medium mixing basin. With a rubber spatula, whisk in the coconut oil, applesauce, agave nectar, and vanilla until the batter is smooth.

Drop the dough onto the baking sheets, about 1 inch apart, using a 14-cup ice-cream scoop or measure. Press the dough to a thickness of 13 inches using the bottom of the measuring cup. Bake for 6 minutes, then rotate the baking sheets and continue baking for another 4 minutes. Allow it cool for 20 minutes on the baking sheets. Spread chocolate sauce on one half of each cookie with a palette knife. Allow 5 minutes for the vanilla icing to set on the other half of each biscuit before serving.

12 servings

Chapter Eleven

COOKIES WITH GINGERBREAD

I admit that sometimes I get so caught up in flavour pairings and texture subtleties that I forget to include the sparkle and excitement in the presentation. My guiding idea has always been simplicity. But then I recall the children! As a result, the heroic Gingerbread Cookies recipe you see before you was created just for them. Gingerbread is a natural canvas for expression. It begs for any kind of icing, can be endlessly adorned, and has just the right amount of spicy flavour to go with a variety of beverages. Serve with your favourite hot chocolate (hint: mine is in my last book!).

213 cup rice flour (brown or white), plus more for dusting

2 cups Bob's Red Mill Gluten-Free All-Purpose Baking Flour

212 cup sugar (vegan)

12 cup arrowroot powder

3 teaspoons ginger powder

2 teaspoons cinnamon powder

xanthan gum, 1 tablespoon

salt (2 tablespoons)

2 teaspoons bicarbonate of soda

14 teaspoon nutmeg, grated

2 cups refined coconut or canola oil, melted

34 cup applesauce, unsweetened

14 teaspoon vanilla extract

13 cup ice water

Decorating using Vanilla Sugar Glaze (optional)

Preheat the oven to 325 degrees Fahrenheit. Set aside 2 rimmed baking sheets lined with parchment paper.

Whisk together 213 cup rice flour, all-purpose flour, sugar, arrowroot, ginger, cinnamon, xanthan gum, salt, baking soda, and nutmeg in a large mixing basin. With a rubber spatula, whisk in the coconut oil, applesauce, and vanilla until a thick dough forms. Stir in the cold water gradually until the dough becomes slightly sticky. Refrigerate for 30 minutes after covering the bowl with plastic wrap.

Dust a clean work area with rice flour, then drop the dough in the centre and roll it about until it is completely covered in flour. More rice flour on the rolling pin. Roll out the dough to a thickness of 14 inches.

Cut out cookies with cookie cutters of your choice and transfer them with a spatula from the work surface to the prepared baking sheets, spacing them about 1 inch apart. Bake for 7 minutes, then rotate the baking sheets and continue baking for another 5 minutes. Allow them cool for 10 minutes on the baking sheets before applying glaze.

36 servings

Chapter Twelve

COOKIES WITH SUGAR

This recipe serves as the foundation for a lifetime of holiday cheer, a blank yet delectable canvas for you and your children to modify till your hearts burst with joy. In terms of texture, I went for a typical crisp, emphasising the flakiness and buttery richness. It's as simple as rolling out the dough. Basically, any flourish you can think of to add to the top—sprinkles? This cookie's density will be enhanced by the addition of Gummi bears and frosting. There's a photo here to show you what you're up against.

214 cup rice flour, plus a little extra for dusting

113 cup sugar (vegan)

14 cup arrowroot powder

1 teaspoon bicarbonate of soda

xanthan gum, 1 teaspoon

1 tblsp. salt

34 cup refined coconut or canola oil, melted

13 cup applesauce, unsweetened

2 tbsp vanilla essence

2 tsp lemon essential oil

13 cup ice water

Decorating using Vanilla Sugar Glaze (optional)

Preheat the oven to 325 degrees Fahrenheit. Set aside 2 rimmed baking sheets lined with parchment paper.

Whisk together the rice flour, sugar, arrowroot, baking soda, xanthan gum, and salt in a medium mixing basin. With a rubber spatula, whisk in the coconut oil, applesauce, vanilla, and lemon extracts until a thick dough forms. Stir in the cold water gradually until the dough becomes slightly sticky. Refrigerate for 30 minutes after covering the bowl with plastic wrap.

Use rice flour to dust a clean work surface. Remove half of the dough from the fridge, set it in the centre, and roll it about until it is completely covered in flour. Rice flour can be used to dust a rolling pin. Roll out the dough to a thickness of 14 inches.

Cut out the cookies with your selected cutters and transfer them with a spatula from the work surface to one of the prepared baking sheets, about 1 inch apart. Rep with the rest of the dough. Bake for 7 minutes, then move the baking sheets and bake for another 5 minutes, or until golden brown. Allow 10 minutes to cool on the baking sheets.

Fill a pastry bag with the sugar glaze and pipe it onto the cookies as desired.

24 servings

Chapter Thirteen

FEELY TOUCHY

Just because I enjoy thin and chewy cookies doesn't imply you will. I experimented and came up with these guidelines to help you fine-tune each cookie recipe to your preferences. Although these changes should work with most BabyCakes cookie recipes, they may not always yield the intended result. Play around, but be cautious and prepared for the mess that may ensue.

This is what you do if this is how you like them...

Cakey and tall

Reduce the vegan sugar by 14 cup and add 12 cup of flour to the batter. The flour will give it height and make it more cake-like, but the reduced sugar will keep it from becoming chewy. Sugar melts, distributes, and caramelises while it cooks, resulting in a compacted and tightly wound cookie.

For That Slightly Undercooked Feel, Soft-Baked

Remove the cookies from the oven 4 minutes before the allotted cooking time and add an additional 14 tsp xanthan gum. Allow the cookies to cool somewhat before eating; otherwise, they may break. You're only left with cookie dough fresh from the fridge!

Hugely Chewy

Prepare for maximum decadence by adding 14 cup vegan sugar and 2 teaspoons heated coconut oil. People, this is not for the faint of heart. When you combine these ingredients, you'll get a candy-like cookie that your oven has never seen before.

Thin as a credit card

14 cup flour is reduced. Bake until the centre is cooked through, about a minute longer than you would with your other batches. If underbaked, the very thin version becomes overly delicate and fragile. When you tap your finger in the centre and it doesn't make a dent, you know they're done.

Chapter Fourteen

SNICKERDOODLES

This is an excellent example of using the illustrious Sugar Cookie as a springboard. You learn to understand its dormant features after enough fiddling with it. What if you asked your brain what would happen if you rolled a butter-taste-based dough in a cinnamon-sugar mixture before baking it? You and your brain are well on your way to total cookie enlightenment if your brain, versed in the ways of the Sugar Cookie, answered that you'd get a beautifully wrinkled explosion of the Snickerdoodle sort.

12 cup vegan sugar plus 113 cup

3 teaspoons cinnamon powder

rice flour, 2 cups

14 cup flaxseed meal

1 teaspoon bicarbonate of soda

xanthan gum, 1 teaspoon

1 tblsp. salt

heated refined coconut oil or canola oil (34 cup plus 2 teaspoons)

12 cup applesauce, unsweetened

2 tbsp vanilla essence

Preheat the oven to 325 degrees Fahrenheit. Set aside 2 rimmed baking sheets lined with parchment paper.

12 cup sugar and 2 teaspoons cinnamon, whisked together in a small basin until evenly combined. Place aside.

Whisk together the 113 cup sugar, flour, flax meal, baking soda, xanthan gum, salt, and the remaining 1 tablespoon cinnamon in a medium mixing basin. With a rubber spatula, combine the coconut oil, applesauce, and vanilla until a thick mixture that resembles wet sand develops. Refrigerate for 1 hour after covering the bowl with plastic wrap.

Drop the dough by the teaspoonful into the cinnamon-sugar mixture and roll it around to coat it all over, working in batches. Place 1 inch apart on the prepared baking pans. To aid spreading, gently push each biscuit with a fork. Bake for 7 minutes, then move the baking sheets and bake for another 7 minutes, or until the edges of the cookies are crisp. Allow to cool for 15 minutes on the baking pans before serving.

36 servings

Chapter Fifteen

MADELEINES

A madeleine is hard to resist. They're attractive, fair, and unmistakably French. These Proustian delicacies have always appealed to the buttery margins of my soul, and they've always been the perfect contrast to my first love, the American chocolate chip cookie, with its rebellious and messy attitude. Plus, I get to use my favourite madeleine tray, which I adore. Get one for yourself and be the talk of the bake sale with your baby girl.

12 cup melted refined coconut or canola oil, plus a little extra for brushing the madeleine trays

114 cup rice flour (white or brown)

1 cup sugar (vegan)

12 cup potato flour

14 cup arrowroot powder

baking powder (212 teaspoons)

1 tblsp. salt

xanthan gum (12 teaspoon)

a quarter teaspoon of baking soda

6 tbsp. applesauce, unsweetened

3 tbsp vanilla essence

12 cup boiling water

12 cup powdered vegan sugar

Preheat the oven to 325 degrees Fahrenheit. Set aside 2 madeleine trays that have been brushed with coconut oil. Using parchment paper, line a baking sheet.

Whisk together the flour, vegan sugar, potato starch, arrowroot, baking powder, salt, xanthan gum, and baking soda in a medium mixing basin. With a rubber spatula, whisk in the 12 cup coconut oil, applesauce, and vanilla until the batter is smooth. Stir in the boiling water gradually until it is all incorporated.

Fill each mould with a rounded tablespoon of batter, carefully spreading it to fill the mould. Bake for 12 minutes, then rotate the trays and bake for another 6 minutes, or until golden brown on top. Remove the trays from the oven and set aside for 15 minutes. Dust the tops of the cooled madeleines with powdered sugar and place them on the prepared baking sheet.

24 servings

COOKIES WITH LACE

Oh, cookies like Stevie Nicks—all twisted around, lovely, and ethereal! A few pointers on how to make this dish your own: Reduce the flour in certain recipes while increasing the sugar in others. You'll learn what proportions make a soft cookie and what proportions produce a chewy cookie by doing so. You'll also learn how to master the crispy edge. Try making a few cookie sandwiches with your favourite glaze or icing in the middle if you're feeling brave—and you probably are by now.

134 cup Bob's Red Mill Gluten-Free All-Purpose Baking Flour

12 cup sugar (vegan)

14 cup arrowroot powder

1 teaspoon bicarbonate of soda

xanthan gum, 1 teaspoon

1 tblsp. salt

1 cup refined coconut or canola oil, melted

12 cup applesauce, unsweetened

2 tbsp vanilla essence

Preheat the oven to 325 degrees Fahrenheit. Set aside 2 rimmed baking sheets lined with parchment paper.

Whisk together the flour, sugar, arrowroot, baking soda, xanthan gum, and salt in a medium mixing basin. Stir in the coconut oil, applesauce, and vanilla with a rubber spatula until completely combined.

1 inch apart, drop the dough by the teaspoonful onto the prepared baking sheets. Bake for 8 minutes, then rotate the pans and bake for another 7 minutes, or until the rims are golden brown and the middle is done. Allow to cool for 15 minutes on the baking pans before serving.

It serves 36 people.

Chapter Sixteen

COOKIES WITH OATMEAL

You would never have seen these in the bakery until Bob's Red Mill came up with a completely inexpensive gluten-free oat. Again, thank everything that is holy for Bob's! These cookies are now in high demand in New York and Los Angeles. If you despise raisins (like I do), try using chocolate chips or dried cherries instead. If you're an oat crazy, you can add up to another 13 cup of oats and be perfectly fine.

134 cup Bob's Red Mill Gluten-Free All-Purpose Baking Flour

1 cup sugar (vegan)

12 cup gluten-free oats from Bob's Red Mill

14 cup flaxseed meal

2 teaspoons cinnamon powder

xanthan gum, 112 tablespoons

1 teaspoon bicarbonate of soda

1 tblsp. salt

1 cup refined coconut or canola oil, melted

12 cup applesauce, unsweetened

2 tbsp vanilla essence

a quarter-cup of raisins

Preheat the oven to 325 degrees Fahrenheit. Set aside 2 rimmed baking sheets lined with parchment paper.

Combine the flour, sugar, oats, flax meal, cinnamon, xanthan gum, baking soda, and salt in a medium mixing bowl. With a rubber spatula, whisk in the coconut oil, applesauce, and vanilla until a thick dough forms. Stir in the raisins until they are uniformly distributed.

1 inch apart, drop the dough by the tablespoonful onto the prepared baking sheets. Bake for 8 minutes, then rotate and bake for another 7 minutes, or until brown. Allow to cool for 15 minutes on the baking pans before serving.

36 servings

Chapter Seventeen

OVERBOARD COOKIE CRAZY FOR VALENTINE'S DAY

I was the odd kid who despised icing and cake in general as a child. But I was willing to put up with any amount of frosting, icing, or other childish suffering if it meant getting one of Mrs. Fields' big Valentine's Day cookies in the window. Obviously, you can make this fanciful concoction with any cookie recipe in this book, but I went ahead and developed a third chocolate chip version (in addition to the bakery standard in the first book and the Chips Ahoy! in this one) to replicate what is found in Mrs. Fields' venerable kitchens. It's large, bold, and buttery all at once. If it helps you visualise it, it's almost like a Toll House cookie.

1 cup heated refined coconut or canola oil, with a little extra for coating the pan

6 tbsp. applesauce, unsweetened

2 tbsp vanilla essence

114 cup sugar (vegan)

1 tblsp. salt

214 cup Bob's Red Mill Gluten-Free All-Purpose Baking Flour

14 cup flaxseed

xanthan gum, 112 tablespoons

1 teaspoon bicarbonate of soda

1 cup gluten-free vegan chocolate chips

4 hours in the refrigerator to chill vanilla icing

Preheat the oven to 325 degrees Fahrenheit. Set aside a 9-inch heart-shaped pan lined with parchment paper and brushed with coconut oil on the bottom and sides.

With a rubber spatula, combine the 1 cup coconut oil, applesauce, vanilla, sugar, and salt in a medium mixing basin. Combine the flour, flax meal, xanthan gum, and baking soda in a separate medium mixing basin. Add the dry ingredients to the wet mixture and stir until a grainy dough forms, using the rubber spatula. Fold the chocolate chips in gently until they're uniformly distributed.

Transfer the dough to the pan and squash it into the mould with the rubber spatula until it is one-third of the way up the sides of the pan. Cook for 22 minutes, or until the middle is fully done. Allow 30 minutes for cooling.

To loosen the sides of the pan, run a knife around the edges. Invert the cookie carefully onto a cutting board. Make sure the cookie is entirely cool before decorating, or the icing will dissolve. Halfway fill the piping bag with frosting. To give a decorative look, pipe along the edges with the piping tip of your choosing. Refrigerate for up to 4 days if stored in an airtight container.

Makes one huge cookie

Chapter Eighteen

WAFERS WITHOUT NILLA

I'm sure I'm not the only one who feels slightly embarrassed about being a Nilla Wafer enthusiast. They're similar to frozen cookie burritos: You don't especially crave them, but they're always there when you're checking out at the supermarket. They are devoured. It's not because they're the only options; it's because they're deceptively tasty. Whatever anyone says, this is a tried-and-true cookie emblem.

oat flour (212 cup)

1 cup sugar (vegan)

2 tblsp. baking powder

1 tblsp. salt

a quarter teaspoon of baking soda

13 cup refined coconut or canola oil, melted

12 cup applesauce, unsweetened

14 teaspoon vanilla extract

Preheat the oven to 325 degrees Fahrenheit. Set aside 2 rimmed baking sheets lined with parchment paper.

Whisk together the flour, sugar, baking powder, salt, and baking soda in a medium mixing basin. With a rubber spatula, whisk in the coconut oil, applesauce, and vanilla until the dough is smooth.

1 inch apart, drop the dough by the teaspoonful onto the prepared baking sheets. Gently press each cookie with the bottom of a measuring cup to flatten it slightly. Bake for 5 minutes, then rotate the pans and bake for another 4 minutes, or until golden brown. Allow to cool for 15 minutes on the baking pans before serving.

48 servings

RECIPES FOR SNACKS

I WAS A VERY HOMELY CHEERLEADER IN MIDDLE SCHOOL. Sure, he's got a lot of spirit, but he's also got gangly appendages, a bowl hairstyle, and can't do back handsprings or even cartwheels. I also have a junk-food addiction and a limited attention span. Even my insatiable desire to wear a cheerleader outfit couldn't save me. So, what's a thin and perennially hungry cheerleader to do but stand on her tiptoes scanning the goodies of the nearby snack bar during her non-cheering game hours? My pantry away from home became the snack bar.

Ultimately, the several hours I spent scouring the various snack sheds of the greater San Diego area's school districts paid off. I was quickly immersed in the complexities of what makes a good snack bar: What about the sweets selection? Are the baked goods motherly gifts or at the very least a well-known and trusted brand? Is there anything resembling a root-beer float on the drink menu? If they have any frozen goods, what are they? Is the pizza cut into squares or slices? Perhaps trivial questions to some. They meant everything to a discerning young lady with $1.50, little interest in sports, and a few hours to kill. In this chapter, I put what I've learned into practise.

Everything from my vegan version of Rice Krispie Blocks to Sno Balls, whoopie pies, and chocolate-dipped frozen bananas can be found here. I also threw in some savoury pizza squares and a sweet-and-spicy popcorn ball, which I've been preparing for weeks. This section's guiding philosophy was nostalgic simplicity, and I'm confident you'll discover more than a few memories of your own while cooking these recipes.

Chapter Nineteen

BLOCKS OF RICE KRISPIE

Beginners and cheapskates beware! This recipe is so simple that you don't even need to turn on the stove (just heat the coconut oil in the microwave!), making it perfect for kids or economical seniors. You can skip the coconut oil if you want to cut the fat in this recipe, but the blocks will not be as buttery. All of the tricks you learned as a kid from your mother apply: To frighten or attract your children, chocolate can be sprinkled on top or throughout, colourful rice cereals can be used, and even dried fruit or nuts can be tossed in.

2 tablespoons heated refined coconut or canola oil, with a little extra for the pan

Ricemellow Crème, 10 oz

1 teaspoon of vanilla extract

1 tblsp. salt

1 box Gluten-Free Brown Rice Crisp Cereal (10 oz.)

Set aside a 9-by-12-inch baking pan brushed with coconut oil.

Blend the Ricemellow Crème, 2 tablespoons coconut oil, vanilla, and salt in a medium mixing bowl and swirl to combine using a rubber spatula. Stir in the rice cereal until all the the Ricemellow Crème is uniformly distributed. Fill the pan halfway with the mixture, cover, and chill for 1 hour. Cut the squares into 3-inch squares.

12 servings

Chapter Twenty

PIE WHOOPIE

I frequently use unrefined sugar to sweeten my cookies because I enjoy the crunch it imparts. Agave nectar, on the other hand, works considerably better in whoopie pies. The reason is simple: Whoopie pies are traditionally made with cookies that are spongy and cake-like in compared to a conventional cookie sandwich. I use Ricemellow Crème, a marshmallow mixture produced by Suzanne's Specialties, for the filling, but Vanilla Icing will work just as well.

12 cup Bob's Red Mill Gluten-Free All-Purpose Baking Flour

12 cup cocoa powder, unsweetened

14 cup arrowroot powder

1 teaspoon bicarbonate of soda

xanthan gum, 1 teaspoon

1 tblsp. salt

1 cup refined coconut or canola oil, melted

agave nectar (23 cup)

12 cup applesauce, unsweetened

2 tbsp vanilla essence

Ricemellow Crème (214 cup)

Preheat the oven to 325 degrees Fahrenheit. Set aside 2 rimmed baking sheets lined with parchment paper.

Combine the flour, cocoa powder, arrowroot, baking soda, xanthan gum, and salt in a medium mixing basin. With a rubber spatula, combine the coconut oil, agave nectar, applesauce, and vanilla until a smooth dough forms.

Using a teaspoon, drop the dough onto the prepared baking sheets, spacing them 112 inches apart. Gently flatten each biscuit with the palm of your hand to help it spread. Bake for 7 minutes, then rotate and bake for another 7 minutes, or until the cookies are firm to the touch and golden brown on the outside. Allow 15 minutes for cooling on the baking sheets.

On the flat side of a cookie, spread 3 tablespoons Ricemellow Crème. Add a second cookie on top. Using the leftover Ricemellow Crème and cookies, repeat the process.

IT'S-IT

My friend Mark introduced me to the city's biggest contribution to the dessert course when I lived in San Francisco: It's-It frozen cookie sandwiches. Two oatmeal cookies with a big scoop of ice cream in between, all thinly coated in semisweet chocolate, are virtually ideal. Mark and I preferred the one with mint ice cream, although you can skip the mint in this recipe if you must. Replace the natural cane sugar with 2/3 cup agave nectar, add an extra 14 cup all-purpose gluten-free flour, remove the chocolate chips, and glaze with Agave-Sweetened Chocolate Glaze to make this agave-sweetened.

2 cups Bob's Red Mill Gluten-Free All-Purpose Baking Flour

1 cup sugar (vegan)

14 cup arrowroot powder

xanthan gum, 112 tablespoons

1 teaspoon bicarbonate of soda

1 tblsp. salt

1 cup refined coconut or canola oil, melted

6 tbsp. applesauce, unsweetened

3 teaspoons peppermint extract

2 tbsp vanilla essence

1 cup gluten-free vegan chocolate chips

2 pints Coconut Bliss mint chip ice cream or your favourite mint ice cream

Chocolate Dipping Sauce with Sugar

Preheat the oven to 325 degrees Fahrenheit. Set aside 2 rimmed baking sheets lined with parchment paper.

Whisk together the flour, sugar, arrowroot, xanthan gum, baking soda, and salt in a medium mixing basin. With a rubber spatula, whisk in the coconut oil, applesauce, peppermint flavouring, and vanilla until the batter is smooth. Add the chocolate chips and mix well.

Drop tablespoonfuls of dough onto baking sheets, leaving 1 inch between cookies. Gently flatten each biscuit with the palm of your hand. Bake for 10 minutes, then rotate and bake for another 4 minutes, or until the cookies are slightly brown. Allow 30 minutes to cool on the baking sheets. If you continue until the cookies have completely cooled, they will break.

In the meantime, make room in the freezer for a baking sheet. Allow the ice cream to soften slightly before making the sandwiches by taking it out of the freezer about 10 minutes before making them. Half of the cookies should be turned upside down. Fill each with 14 cup ice cream, then top with the remaining cookies. Dip each sandwich halfway or completely into the chocolate sauce with chopsticks or two forks. Place the remaining sandwiches on a baking sheet and repeat. Freeze the cookies for about 30 minutes, or until the chocolate coating has hardened. Remove the sandwiches from the freezer and wrap each one in a double layer of plastic wrap.

12 to 15 ice cream sandwich sandwiches

Chapter Twenty-one

S'MORES

This recipe will give you buttery, crunchy graham crackers, which is just how I like them. In fact, this graham cracker is so rich that you might want to double the recipe to have leftovers on purpose. These can be used for a lot of different things. For example, piecrust! For two, donut toppings!

CRACKERS FOR GRAHAMS

1 cup vegan sugar + 13 cup sprinkling sugar

3 teaspoons cinnamon powder

12 cup rice flour for dusting additional 112 cup rice flour

12 cup Bob's Red Mill Gluten-Free All-Purpose Baking Flour

2 tablespoons ginger powder

xanthan gum, 1 teaspoon

1 tblsp. salt

34 cup refined coconut or canola oil warmed, plus 14 cup for brushing

agave nectar (14 cup)

1 teaspoon of vanilla extract

12 cup ice water

FOR THE COMPLETION

Ricemellow Crème, 2 cups

1 batch Sugar-Sweetened Chocolate Dipping Sauce or Agave-Sweetened Chocolate Glaze (or a little less)

Preheat the oven to 325 degrees Fahrenheit. Set aside two rimmed baking sheets lined with parchment paper.

13 cup vegan sugar and 1 tablespoon cinnamon, whisked together in a small dish. Place aside.

Whisk together the 112 cup rice flour, all-purpose flour, remaining sugar and cinnamon, ginger, xanthan gum, and salt in a medium basin. With a rubber spatula, combine the 34 cup coconut oil, agave nectar, and vanilla until a thick dough forms. Slowly drizzle in the cold water, mixing until the dough becomes slightly sticky. Refrigerate for 30 minutes after wrapping in plastic wrap.

Place the dough in the centre of a clean work surface dusted with the majority of the remaining 12 cup rice flour. Roll the dough in rice flour until it is completely covered. Roll out the dough to a thickness of 14 inches using a rolling pin dusted with rice flour. Cut the dough into 3-inch squares with a knife. Place the squares on the baking sheets, approximately an inch apart. Brush the remaining 14 cup coconut oil over the squares, then sprinkle each with 34 teaspoon of the cinnamon-sugar mixture. Bake for 10 minutes, then rotate and bake for another 5 minutes, or until the crackers are deep golden. Allow 10 minutes to cool on the baking sheets.

Half of the graham crackers should be turned upside down. Top each graham cracker with 2 heaping tablespoons Ricemellow Crème, 114 teaspoons chocolate sauce, and a second graham cracker.

18 servings

Chapter Twenty-two

BALLS OF SNO

Sno Balls, like bubble-gum ice cream, were one of those grocery-store things I wanted as a child. I only knew they looked like Barbie food, which was exactly what I wanted and required. Then I tried another. Absolutely horrible. That's bad. I couldn't understand how something so lovely could taste so bad. Then, when it came time to write this book, I decided that something so cute didn't have to taste so awful. As a result, I reworked them. I discovered a new bakery favourite in the process. Furthermore, you get two recipes in the process of creating a batch of them; check out the Bread Pudding recipe for an example of what you can do with the wasted portion of a cupcake.

1 cup coconut (unsweetened)

12 teaspoons natural red food colouring from India Tree

34 cup rice flour (white or brown)

12 cup flour made from sorghum

12 cup potato flour

14 cup arrowroot powder

1 tablespoon powdered sugar

a quarter teaspoon of baking soda

xanthan gum (12 teaspoon)

1 tblsp. salt

agave nectar (23 cup)

12 cup refined coconut or canola oil, melted

13 cup applesauce, unsweetened

14 teaspoon vanilla extract

1 teaspoon lemon essential oil

12 cup boiling water

Ricemellow Crème 112 cup

Preheat the oven to 325 degrees Fahrenheit. Set aside a muffin tray lined with cupcake liners.

Toss the coconut with the red food colouring in a small basin with your hands until the flakes are consistently coloured. If you want a brighter pink, add a little extra food colouring. Place aside.

Whisk together the flours, potato starch, arrowroot, baking powder, baking soda, xanthan gum, and salt in a medium mixing basin. With a rubber spatula, combine the agave nectar, coconut oil, applesauce, vanilla, and lemon extract until the batter is smooth. Mix in the boiling water until it is completely incorporated.

Divide the batter amongst the baking cups using a 12-cup measure. Bake for 14 minutes, then rotate and bake for another 14 minutes, or until the cupcakes are gently brown on the exterior and a toothpick inserted in the centre comes out clean. Allow 30 minutes in the tin to cool.

Remove the cupcake liners from each one. Remove the bottom third of the cupcake and save it for another time. Hollow out the remaining piece of the cupcakes with a spoon and fill each with 1 tablespoon Ricemellow Crème. Top each snowball with an additional 2 tablespoons crème and roll in the pink coconut.

12 servings

Chapter Twenty-three

TIPS

CHOCOLATE-DIPPED BANANAS, FROZEN

Even though the Sugar-Sweetened Chocolate Dipping Sauce might stiffen up a little better in the freezer than the alternative, you'll notice that this recipe doesn't call for it. Instead, I opt for the agave-sweetened version since I don't see the point in coating a perfectly nutritional snack with vegan sugar when an agave-sweetened alternative is available.

6 peeled bananas

Chocolate Glaze with Agave.

12 sticks of popsicle

TOPPINGS RECOMMENDED

Granola

Coconut Toasted

Crumbled Graham crackers

Set aside a rimmed baking sheet lined with parchment paper.

Remove the tips from each banana and slice it in half before placing it on the baking sheet. Place each in the freezer for 20 minutes after inserting a Popsicle stick into the broad end. Dip each banana in chocolate glaze, then roll in your preferred topping. Return the bananas to the baking sheet and freeze for another 45 minutes.

12 servings

Chapter Twenty-four

ROYALE BANANA

Raw bananas taste too healthy for a sundae surrounded by all that other sweet mayhem, therefore I'm not a fan of the traditional banana split. So I add some love and caramelise the bananas, which turns them into a deeply textured miracle with a buttery flavour not found in your average banana split.

2 peeled ripe bananas

3 tablespoons refined coconut or canola oil, melted

1 tablespoon sugar (vegan)

1 pint coconut bliss brand vegan gluten-free vanilla ice cream

Ricemellow Crème (12 cup)

1 cup chocolate glaze sweetened with agave

13 cup almonds, sliced (optional)

4 pitted red cherries

Cut the bananas in half lengthwise, then crosswise into thirds. Heat the coconut oil in a medium skillet over medium heat until it is hot, about 45 seconds. Stir in the sugar and bananas with a wooden spoon until they are caramelised, being careful not to break up the bananas.

In each of the four dessert bowls, place 1 heaping scoop of ice cream. Divide the banana mixture into the bowls and top with 2 tablespoons Ricemellow Crème. Drizzle 14 cup chocolate glaze over each. If using, sprinkle with almonds and finish with a cherry.

Approximately 4 sundaes

Chapter Twenty-five

BALLS OF SWEET AND SPICY POPCORN

This is one of my all-time favourite snacks—a perfectly balanced blend of ingredients. Don't put these in a big bowl next to the couch and settle down for a reality-TV marathon while pretending to write a cookbook as I did on a windy, rainy spring day. I guarantee you will lose the productivity struggle. Instead, create a large quantity and divide the balls into separate airtight sandwich bags for easy consumption during the week.

2 cups hulled pumpkin seeds or almond slivers

12 cups fresh popped popcorn or 3 3.5-ounce bags natural microwave popcorn

agave nectar (2 cups)

12 gallon coconut milk

2 tbsp. melted refined coconut or canola oil, plus a little extra chevalier

1 teaspoon essence of vanilla

12 tablespoons salt

12 teaspoon cinnamon powder

12 teaspoon chilli powder

Preheat the oven to 350 degrees Fahrenheit. Using parchment paper, line a rimmed baking sheet.

Bake the pumpkin seeds or almonds in a single layer on the baking sheet for 10 minutes, stirring once, or until beautifully toasted. Place in a large heat-resistant bowl and put aside. Transfer the popcorn to the bowl after popping it according to the package directions. Toss the popcorn with the seeds or nuts until everything is evenly distributed. Place aside.

In a medium saucepan, combine the agave nectar and 12 cup water and bring to a boil over medium heat, stirring every other minute to prevent the mixture from sticking to the pan. Reduce the heat to low and cook for another 10 minutes, or until the liquid acquires a rich caramel colour. Remove the pan from the heat and set aside for 1 minute. Add the coconut milk, 2 tablespoons coconut oil, vanilla, salt, cinnamon, and cayenne pepper while whisking vigorously until the caramel is smooth. Allow 1 minute to cool before pouring the caramel over the popcorn and stirring until evenly coated. Refrigerate the mixture for at least 20 minutes.

Wear hygienic rubber gloves and a dime-sized glob of coconut oil in one hand's palm. Form the popcorn mixture into 3-inch balls by rubbing your hands together until your palms are lightly coated.

20 servings

TOMATO SQUARE-PAN PIZZA

Have you noticed how many gluten-free pizza parlours have recently opened in major cities? I have, and pizza excites me tremendously! My version's end result is straightforward and traditional—tomatoes, garlic, and a pinch of basil on top of a thin crust—even though the crust's directions require some attention. Above all, make certain to purchase the best tomatoes you can find. If you must (as I frequently do), sprinkle some cheese on top and pile on as many vegetables as you want—just be sure to roll your dough a little thicker to support the extra weight. I've also included a tried-and-true tomato sauce for the purists among you.

DUE TO THE CRUST

12 cup Bob's Red Mill Gluten-Free All-Purpose Baking Flour

12 cup rice flour (brown)

12 cup flour made from sorghum

1 tablespoon powdered sugar

1 tblsp. salt

xanthan gum (12 teaspoon)

6 tablespoons refined coconut or canola oil, melted

agave nectar (1 tablespoon)

1 minced garlic clove

1 cup of iced water

FOR THE FINISHING

4 tablespoons refined coconut oil, canola oil, or extra virgin olive oil, melted

5 finely sliced Roma tomatoes

4 minced garlic cloves

salt (2 tablespoons)

12 tsp. chilli flakes

12 cup cornmeal (to dust)

a handful of basil leaves torn

Preheat the oven to 350 degrees Fahrenheit. Set aside a rimmed baking sheet lined with parchment paper.

To prepare the crust, whisk together the flours, baking powder, salt, and xanthan gum in a medium mixing basin. With a rubber spatula, combine the coconut oil, agave nectar, garlic, and cold water until a thick dough forms. Refrigerate the dough for 20 minutes after wrapping it in plastic wrap.

To prepare the topping, put 1 tablespoon coconut oil, tomatoes, garlic, salt, and chilli flakes in a medium mixing bowl and toss to incorporate. Place aside.

Cornmeal should be used to dust a clean work surface. Place the dough on top and sprinkle some of the cornmeal on top. Make a 14-inch-thick rectangle out of the dough. Trim any excess dough from the edges of the dough before transferring it to the prepared baking sheet. Brush the remaining 3 tablespoons coconut oil over the dough. Bake for 15 minutes, or until brown. Remove the pan from the oven and top with the tomato mixture. Garnish with basil leaves. Bake for another 15 minutes or until the vegetables are tender. Cut the dough into nine squares.

Approximately 9 squares

Chapter Twenty-six

STRAWS OF CHEESE

This one gets a higher rating on the BabyCakes Piece of Cake scale since it necessitates pastry assembly, which always adds to the complexity. It may take a little while for you sophomores to get your stride, and your first few straws may most likely resemble craggy witch fingers, but perseverance will pay off. When it does, you should throw a dinner party and serve these by the pint.

12 cup brown rice flour plus 34 cup brown rice flour

12 cup Bob's Red Mill Gluten-Free All-Purpose Baking Flour

3 tablespoons cornmeal

14 cup arrowroot powder

1 tablespoon powdered sugar

xanthan gum, 112 tablespoons

1 tblsp. salt

13 cup refined coconut or canola oil, melted

314 cup vegan gluten-free cheese

agave nectar (14 cup)

Preheat the oven to 325 degrees Fahrenheit. Set aside 2 rimmed baking sheets lined with parchment paper.

Whisk together the 34 cup rice flour, all-purpose flour, cornmeal, arrowroot, baking powder, xanthan gum, and salt in a medium basin. Stir in the coconut oil, 114 cups of cheese, and the agave nectar (the mixture will be very dry). Slowly drizzle in up to a third of a cup of water until the dough becomes sticky. The dough should be divided in half.

Place half of the dough on a clean work area and dust with the remaining 14 cup rice flour. Sprinkle more rice flour on top of the dough and roll it out into a 14-inch-thick rectangle. Half of the rectangle should be covered in cheese. Place the naked dough on top, sandwiching the cheese between two layers of dough. Pinch the open edges of the dough together to make 4-inch-long 1-inch-wide strips. Place on one of the baking sheets that has been prepped. Rep with the rest of the dough. On top of the strips, sprinkle the remaining cheese.

Bake for 10 minutes, rotate, then bake for another 8 minutes or until the cheese straws are golden brown.

24 servings

TOMATO SAUCE WHEN I DIP, YOU DIP, WE DIP

It's simple to make your own tomato-based sauce to dip your cheese straws in or spread on your pizza. We normally throw something together at the bakery with any leftover vegetables and scraps we have. The foundation, on the other hand, looks like this.

1 full peeled 12-ounce tomato can

2 cloves garlic

1 cup sliced zucchini

Basil leaves, a small handful

12 cup olives, pitted

1 tblsp. salt

1 teaspoon cayenne pepper

3 tablespoons extra virgin olive oil or melted coconut oil

Simply combine all ingredients in a food processor and pulse until smooth. Keep the pizza thick in the recipe. Blend the cheese sticks until they resemble your favourite salsa.

212 cup yield

Chapter Twenty-seven

HAMENTASCHEN

I admit that the first time a customer asked for hamentaschen, I had to go to a nearby kosher bakery to find out what they were talking about. However, I quickly recognised them and fell in love with every variation of light pastry loaded with jam. In the centre, you can use any preserve or jam you choose, but I've given a recipe for my favourite blackberry filling. With the exception of raspberries, which are quite liquid and don't thicken up very well, you can easily substitute another berry.

JAM WITH BLACKBERRIES

blackberries, 2 quarts

agave nectar (3 cups)

lemon juice, 3 teaspoons

1 tsp arrowroot powder

12 cup opium poppy seeds

Dough for Gluten-Free Pastries

In a large saucepan, combine the blackberries, agave nectar, lemon juice, arrowroot, and poppy seeds. Bring to a boil, then lower to a low heat. Allow to cook for 45 minutes, uncovered, stirring periodically. Allow to cool before serving. Fill an airtight container halfway with jam.

Preheat the oven to 325 degrees Fahrenheit. Set aside 2 rimmed baking sheets lined with parchment paper.

Roll out the dough to a thickness of 14 inches on a clean work surface. Cut the dough into rounds with a 2-inch biscuit cutter. Fill the middle of each circle with a tablespoon of jam filling. To make a perfect triangle, find three independent, equidistant places on the perimeter of the rounds. Grab the dough at these three points and draw it up around the filling one at a time to make a tent, pinching the points and seams together while leaving a little of the filling exposed (as pictured).

Bake for 15 minutes on the prepared baking pans, then rotate and bake for another 7 minutes, or until the edges are golden. Remove from the oven and set aside for 10 minutes on the baking sheets.

30 servings

Chapter Twenty-eight

RUGALACH

This is another Jewish recipe that quickly became a bakery classic. I don't know about you, but I'm a sucker for folded pastry in any form. If you asked me to do something all day, I would pull away the layers and investigate and enjoy the various textures inside. Normally, rugalach recipes call for nuts, but I left them out in honour of those who suffer from allergies.

34 cup sugar (vegan)

2 tablespoons cinnamon powder

1 tbsp agave nectar plus 13 cup

2 tablespoons refined coconut or canola oil, melted

a quarter cup of rice flour

Dough for Gluten-Free Pastries

1 cup apricot preserves (bought or homemade) or blackberry jam

1 cup chopped raisins

walnuts, 1 cup (optional)

Preheat the oven to 350 degrees Fahrenheit. Set aside 2 rimmed baking sheets lined with parchment paper.

Set aside 12 cup of the sugar and the cinnamon in a small mixing dish. In a separate small bowl, add the agave nectar and coconut oil and stir until fully blended. Place aside.

Use the rice flour to dust a clean work area and a rolling pin. Roll out about a quarter of the dough onto the work surface into a 14-inch-thick rectangle. Place the dough on a piece of parchment and chill while you roll out the remaining dough in the same manner. Place the second dough rectangle in the fridge to chill.

Place 1 chilled dough part on the work surface, long side facing you. Spread ¼ cup of the preserves or jam onto the dough. 14 cup raisins, 14 cup walnuts (if using), and 2 teaspoons cinnamon-sugar mixture should be sprinkled over it. Form a tight log out of the dough. Place it on a baking sheet and crimp the ends together. Repeat with the remaining dough, spacing the logs 1 inch apart on one of the baking sheets that has been prepared. Brush the agave mixture on the logs and finish with the leftover cinnamon sugar. Make 34-inch-deep crosswise slashes in the dough at 1-inch intervals with a sharp knife, being careful not to cut through to the bottom. Rep with the rest of the dough.

Bake for 15 minutes, then rotate and bake for an additional 10 minutes, or until golden brown. Let stand on the baking sheets for 20 minutes, then transfer the logs to a cutting board and slice the cookies all the way through.

40 servings

Chapter Twenty-nine

SODA BREAD FROM IRELAND

When I told my brothers and sisters that I was including Irish soda bread in this cookbook, they were horrified. I'm not sure I blame them. When we visited Grandma McKenna after church, she would have us do it as a punishment for disrupting her Sunday afternoon cleaning spree. Grandma would ask him if he wanted some sweets, and if he responded yes, she'd seat him down with a thick slice of Irish soda bread, according to my brother Bill. "Put some butter on it!" she would say in response to complaints, according to my brother Frank. Instead, I chose to just modernise this classic snack so that it can compete with the growth of delicate tastebuds.

13 quart rice milk

apple cider vinegar, 1 tablespoon

14 cup oat flour for dusting, plus 314 cup oat flour

12 c. raisins

14 cup currants, dry

caraway seeds, 3 tablespoons

2 tblsp. baking powder

xanthan gum, 1 teaspoon

¾ teaspoon salt

a quarter teaspoon of baking soda

14 cup refined coconut or canola oil, melted

agave nectar (2 teaspoons)

Preheat the oven to 350 degrees Fahrenheit. Set aside a rimmed baking sheet lined with parchment paper.

Combine the rice milk and vinegar in a small bowl. Place aside.

Combine the flour, raisins, currants, caraway seeds, baking powder, xanthan gum, salt, and baking soda in a medium mixing basin. With a rubber spatula, stir in the coconut oil, agave nectar, and rice-milk mixture until a sticky dough forms.

Half of the reserved flour should be sprinkled on the baking sheet. Roll the dough into a ball and dust with the remaining flour. Make a 14-inch deep incision across the top of the bread using a sharp knife.

Bake for 20 minutes, then rotate and bake for another 20 minutes, or until a toothpick inserted in the centre comes out clean. If the bottom of the loaf sounds hollow when tapped, it's done. Allow to cool on a rack.

This recipe makes one 5-inch circular loaf.

CPSIA information can be obtained
at www.ICGtesting.com
Printed in the USA
BVHW011419090822
644143BV00007B/455